101
Simple Steps
to
Radiant Health

by
Logan Christopher

DISCLAIMER

The advice contained within this book is for educational purposes only and is not intended for medical purposes. Please consult your physician before engaging in any of the ideas found in these pages.

The author and publisher of this book are not responsible in any manner whatsoever for the use, misuse or dis-use of the information presented here.

Dedication

To all the sources and people who have helped me in learning, using and now teaching the information here.

And most of all to my much loved and departed mother. May this book help people avoid the hell you went through.

benefits feel free to discard the technique. More often than not the small tips would be hard to judge on an individual basis. The can have subtle effect while others will have a profound effect. Let it be known that the cumulative effect of many of them can be seen and felt with definiteness.

With this collection of knowledge you can add years to your life and life to your years.

In Health,
Logan Christopher

1
Breathe From Your Diaphragm

Watch a baby breathe. How do they do it? Each and every breathe goes deep into the diaphragm so that the stomach rises and falls. Many people as they grow up lose their ability to breathe in this manner through dis-use. But it can be regained. By employing diaphragmatic breathing all day long you'll get more oxygen into your system. Oxygen is good. In fact all bad bacteria cannot survive in an oxygen rich environment. In the beginning, just focus on breathing as deep into your body as possible, when you are practicing the other deep breathing exercises from the following tips. As you continue this practice you'll find that you naturally begin to breathe deeply all the time.

2
<u>Breathe Through Your Nose</u>

Breathing can be done through the mouth and through the nose. However, using your nose is the superior way to go. Inside the nose is a filtration system that is meant to keep out harmful particles. You forgo this defense system every time you breathe through the mouth. Breathing through the mouth is usually used to get more air into the body. By learning how to breathe deep you'll not need to open your mouth in 99% of situations. Intense exercise being the one big exception. Because you need more oxygen you must open your mouth. That is fine in this case but as you go through your average day breathing through your nose is preferred.

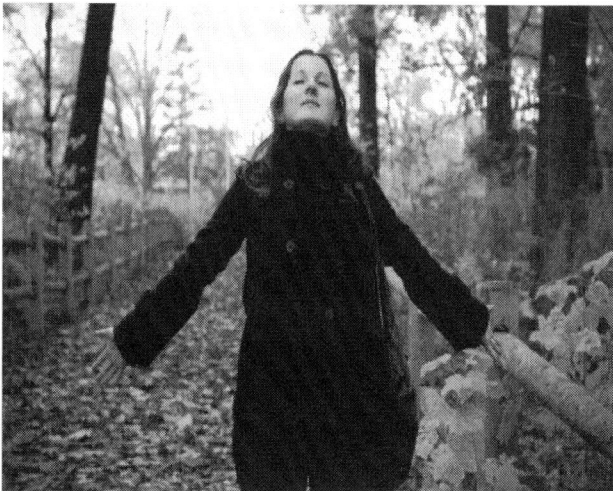

3
Sleep With Open Windows

We spend about a third of our life sleeping. That is a significant portion of everyday in this state. Breathing does not stop when you sleep (and if it does then you've got some bigger problems to worry about). You won't be able to consciously improve your breathing then but you can improve the quality of air you get during that time. Most people close the windows to keep the cold out. Instead grab another blanket and let the air in. You want the fresh air for you to breathe rather than the stagnant air you would be taking in. And whenever you're in doors, to the best of your ability you should keep the windows open to keep the fresh air circulating.

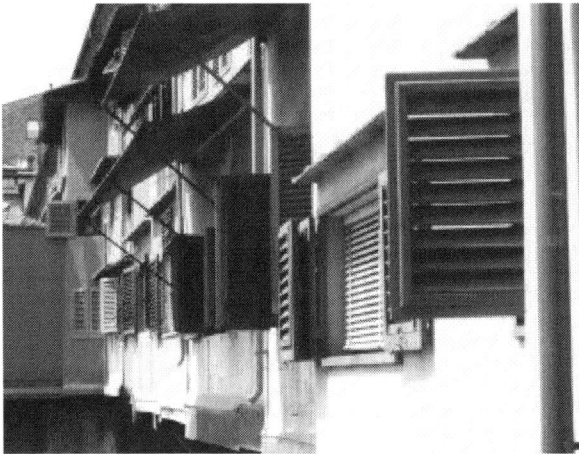

4
Breathing Before Sleeping

Right before you go to bed is a prime time to take a few deep breaths. You can review you day in your mind or look at what you'll be doing tomorrow. You can think about how you'll be waking up rejuvenated. Just take ten deep breaths. You may find you'll breathe better during your sleep and that the quality is improved. Plus you're likely to fall asleep faster.

5
Breathing Before Arising

Right when you wake up in the morning is another prime time to get some deep breathing exercises in. You can use the bathroom and drink some water first, but take a few minutes to fill your lungs with life-giving air. Especially if you go outside. In the early mornings the air outside just seems fresher. Take advantage of this time.

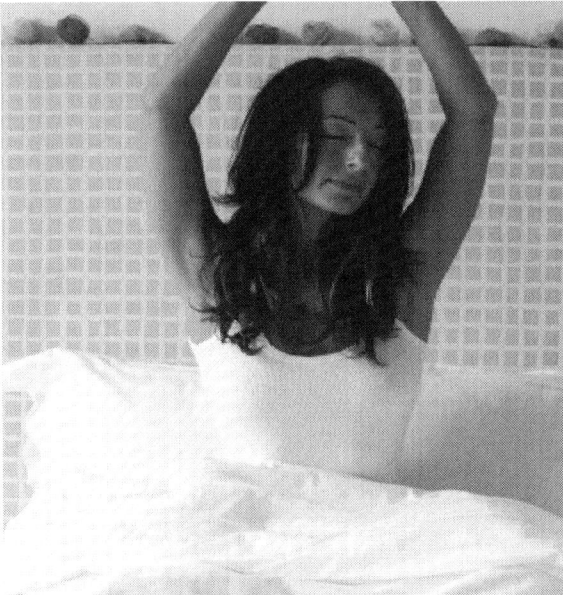

6
<u>Drink A Lot Of Water</u>

There is much more to water then just drinking enough of it but that will be covered later. That being said drinking enough water is very important. Over 75% of people are chronically dehydrated. Virtually every bodily process requires water. And the big problem is that you're likely to mistake thirst for hunger. How much do you need to drink? It will depend on several factors. Size and weight are the first ones. Larger individuals need more. The more active you are, especially if the activity causes you to sweat, then you will need to replace that water. It also depends on the rest of your diet. A bare minimum of a half gallon a day is required. For most people a full gallon is the goal to shoot for. Take a challenge to down a full gallon each day for a week and see how you feel.

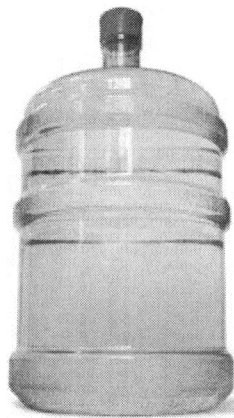

7
Drink First Thing In The Morning

You have just gone approximately eight hours without taking in any water. You may be sleeping but your body still uses up water. As soon as you get out of bed it is important to replenish what you have lost. Drink a large amount of water to start your day. Even as much as a quart or liter. Do you need to drink this much? Maybe, maybe not. Experiment for yourself. But at least get a tall glass in.

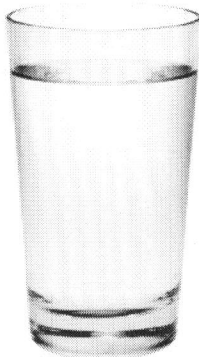

8
Drink Before Retiring At Night

Prepare yourself for the eight hour drought you are about to go through. You do not need to drink a huge amount at this time as most likely you do not want to have to use the bathroom several times at night. Eight ounces would work well in most cases. Just enough to help the body do its work at night. This will depend on your thirst as well as how hydrated you stayed during the day.

9
Do Not Drink With Your Meals

Taking in water or most liquids serves to dilute your digestive juices in most cases. (Certain liquids may help.) It further complicates the work your body must do to digest food. As a general rule you should not drink for 15 minutes before a meal and for at least an hour after a meal. This will depend also on the size and content of the meal. The important thing is to not need liquid to wash down any food you have eaten. If you need that then pay attention to tip number 12.

10
Add Lemon To Your Water

By adding lemon to your water you are making it more hydrating. Lemon juice in and of itself is very beneficial. The acidic nature of the lemon makes the body go into an alkaline reaction. Also some people do not enjoy the taste of regular water. By adding lemon you are adding some flavor. I personally enjoy squeezing a whole lemon or lime into my morning water everyday.

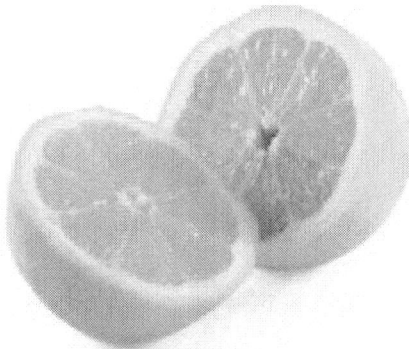

11
<u>Drink High Quality Water</u>

Everyone knows that you need to drink a lot of water, whether they do it or not. But it may be more important to get the best quality water. Water is actually quite complex and its not all created equal. Besides the pollutants found in almost all tap water, the water's structure may not be in the best bio-available form. Try to avoid bottled water as its expensive and wasteful for the environment. Instead get a high quality filter as well as a method to structure the water (its best form is hexagonal). This will allow the water to penetrate deeper into the body and cells allowing true hydration on all levels. There are many methods, some better than others, for accomplishing this goal. The water technologies and filtration I currently use are available at www.legendarystrength.com/go/watertech

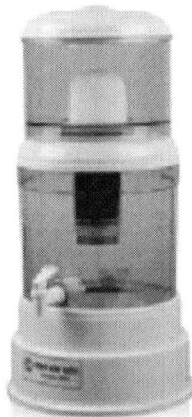

12
Chewing Your Food

If you want to get more nutritional value from the food you already eat its as simple as chewing it more while it's in your mouth. While the stomach has various acids and enzymes used to break down food it has no teeth that can be used manually to do the job. Make sure you chew each mouthful at the very least 20 times (this depends on the type of food). The rule of thumb is to chew everything up into a fine paste or liquid before swallowing. This goes hand in hand with the next point.

13
Pay Attention To Eating

Here is a simple tip that will help you get more enjoyment out of food and will make chewing it much easier. When you eat, eat and do nothing else. With today's multitasking society it can be hard to sit down and enjoy a meal without working, watching TV, or anything else. Have you ever ate a meal while doing something else and not even tasted it or remember doing it? Well now it's time to enjoy your food. This will help you to get in touch with your hunger and satiation levels so that you eat the proper amount instead of just shoveling food in mindlessly.

14
What Macro-Nutrient Fuels You Best?

Every person is different. This includes when it comes to nutrition. This is one of the main reason some diets work well for certain people and not for others. If you're fueled best from carbohydrates and you go on a low-carb diet you'll be miserable. For me personally, fat is the best fuel therefore my diet is made up of 40-50% fat. It works for me. Find which of the three macro-nutrients (fat, carbohydrate, or protein) fuels you best and work from there. For most people eating balanced meals will work best, although that balance will probably not be equal thirds. If you are unaware of your best fuel, to experiment start your morning off by enjoying a meal of only one macro-nutrient, or close to it. See how this works for you.

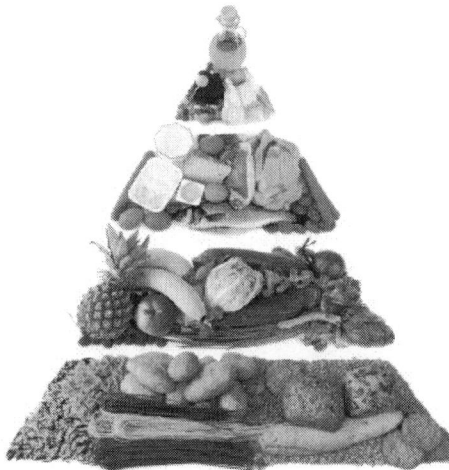

15
When To Eat?

Just like macro-nutrients can work different for different people, different times to eat are the same. Experiment with the timing of your meals. A big large breakfast may not be best for you, or maybe it is. Do you need lunch? Should you have meals and snacks throughout the day or are you better suited to eating one large meal at night? Maybe the standard, three square meals does work. Find out what works for you. And don't expect it to be the same for all time.

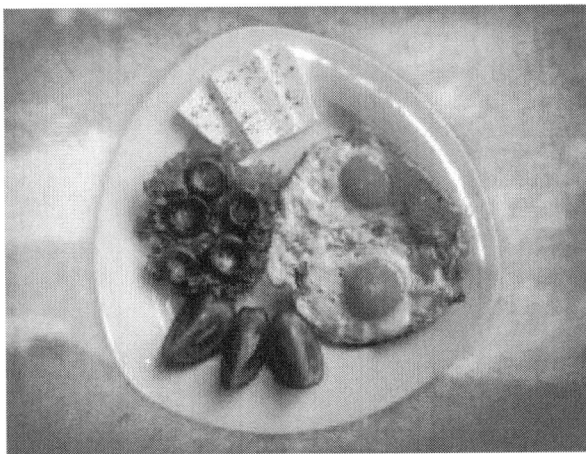

16

Eat Organic

There are two main health reasons to eat organic. First off, organic foods are not sprayed with poisons to combat various other creatures from eating them. If these kill other things that eat them, do you think they're good for you? And have you ever seen the pictures of people in full biohazard suits spraying fields of crops? They need that protection from the chemicals yet we eat it. Doesn't seem right. And if you only get organic fruits and vegetables you're missing a key point. Its even more important in animal products as all those harmful chemicals are concentrated up into animals who eat the same stuff. Secondly, organic foods contain more nutrition with much higher amounts of vitamins and minerals. By doing some research you can find which foods are better or worse off if organic or conventional. If you're serious about your health this is a must.

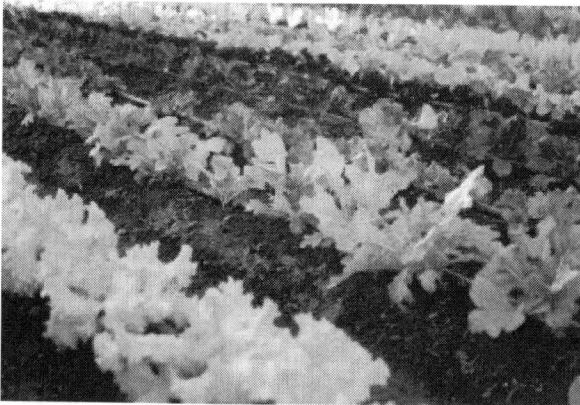

17
<u>*Eat When Hungry*</u>

The average person these days is really out of tune with their hunger. They may say they're starving when they haven't eaten in a couple hours, yet they've never felt true hunger. And hopefully you'll never have to. The point is, being out of touch with hunger causes you to eat more than necessary and likely worse foods then necessary. Instead, what if you only ate when hungry and only as much as was needed to satiate that hunger. The following tips should help you to get better in tune.

18
Fermented Foods

Fermented foods and the probiotics, or helpful bacteria, they contain are an essential piece of good health. Most people's diets are completely devoid of these things, and as a result their intestinal flora is in bad shape. But a healthy gut means a healthy body. Add more and more of these foods into your daily diet; sauerkraut, kombucha, apple cider vinegar, yogurt, raw milk, kefir and others. (Note that some of these products come in live forms and others have been heated which will kill off all probiotics. Know the difference.) More research is coming out all the time pointing to this as one of the most important factors in great health, as this helpful bacteria does much more than help with digestion.

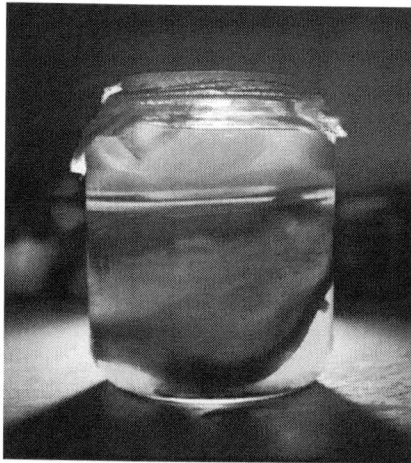

19
Enjoy Spicy Food

While not everyone enjoys it there are benefits to eating spicy food. They are high in anti-oxidants and have anti-inflammatory properties (though it may feel otherwise if you go too spicy). It causes an increase of circulation and in general opens the body up. Start with what you can and overtime your capacity and enjoyment of hot and spicy foods will increase. That being said do not go overboard. I once ate a habenero pepper by itself and had to lie down for some time afterward. Moderation is key.

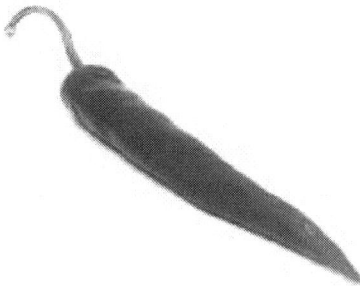

20
Eat Variety Of Foods

We're not meant to eat the same thing all the time. Its good to have daily habits and its certainly easier but there needs to be variation in your diet. Eat seasonal fruits and vegetables as a starting point. Always look for new foods to try out. You may just find the best food in the world if you do. On top of this do variations on the things you regularly eat. Different spices or side dishes. Different foods in the mix for smoothies or juices.

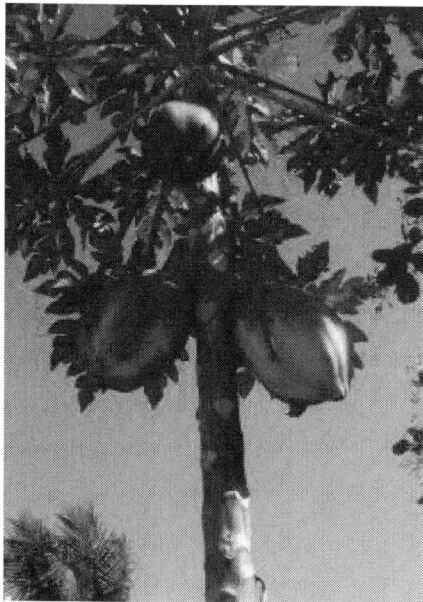

21
Eat Fruit Or Vegetables Before Meals

Living foods have enzymes that help break down the food for digestion. When a food is cooked these enzymes are cooked as well. In fact, they're among the first things to go when any food is heated. If you don't get these with your food your body must use its own limited supply. You don't have to eliminate cooked food altogether unless you want to become a raw foodist. But realize that these enzymes are important. So before any meal eat something that has them intact. An orange or apple before breakfast is great. And a salad before dinner. Make this a regular habit.

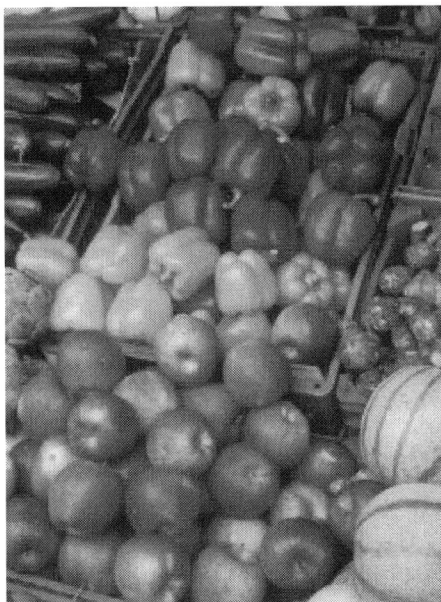

22
<u>Salad Everyday</u>

If there is one thing most people need to eat more of its leafy green vegetables. Don't tell me you don't like the taste, get over it and soon you'll find you do. (Check out tip 24 for a method of overcoming this.) Make it a habit to eat a medium to large salad everyday. This gives you fiber, chlorophyll and several other benefits. Watch what you put on it though, especially the salad dressing. I enjoy just using olive oil, though do on occasions have 'dry' salads.

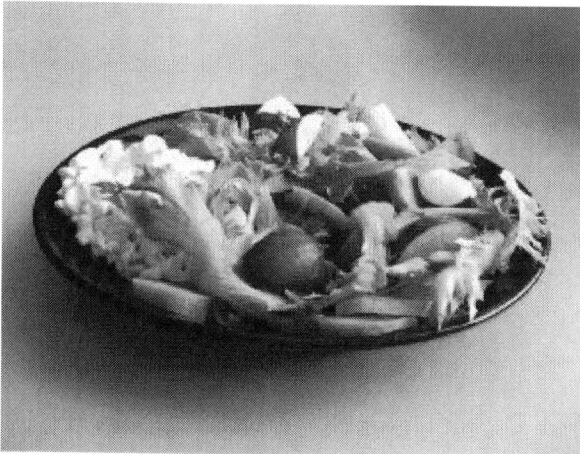

23

Raw Food

If you eat cooked food your body attacks it with the white blood cells as if it was an invading virus or other invader. It takes at least 50% raw food for this not to happen. Having a high amount of raw food in your diet gives you more of what your body needs as cooking often damages or degrades the quality of all the nutrition found within food. In fact cooking will often cause chemical alterations in the food. There are some people who even eat only 100% raw food at all times. While this may not be right for everyone having more raw food in your diet most likely is. As you become healthier you'll find this number goes up overtime. I would encourage you to have your diet be supplied by at least 50% raw food. For those looking to lose weight, going in this direction is an easy way to start shedding those pounds, as overeating raw foods, especially vegetables is hard to do. For more information I highly recommend <u>The Sunfood Diet Success System</u> by David Wolfe.

24
Juicing

Juicing fruits and vegetables is a fast, fun and delicious way to get a high amount of nutrition into your body. It can also help to acclimate your taste buds to various fruits and vegetables. Drinking the juice will get you use to the taste without messing with the texture. After awhile you'll find you don't mind or even enjoy eating them. You can make all kinds of juice so be sure to experiment with different combinations. I would encourage you to use more vegetables than fruits as too much sugar (from apples or carrots for instance) without any fiber may cause your blood sugar to increase. Work with a base of celery, cucumber, and leafy greens. Add the others to taste.

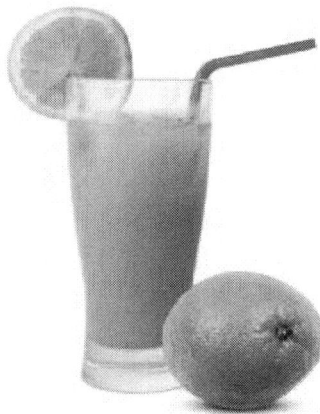

25
Liquefy Food

Not all technology is bad or harmful. Much of it can be used to improve our lives and our health. Blenders and juicers are two such items. Digestion is one of the most energy intensive processes of the body. Getting vital enzymes and probiotics are two important pieces which have already been described. On top of that you can make the job easier by breaking down the food into an easily digestible form. Juicing has already been discussed. But you can also blend. By doing this you break down the structure into something much smaller than you likely would with your teeth. This makes the stomach's job much easier. You can also combine a wide variety of foods, including superfoods, that we'll be getting to shortly for a highly nutritious, highly digestible meal. Even though it's liquefied don't just gulp it down. Make sure to swish it around the mouth (and chew if necessary) to mix in the saliva.

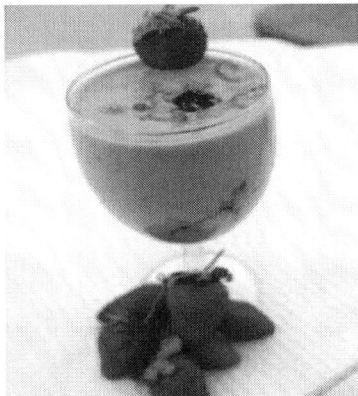

26
Cold-Stoppers

There are certain foods that have strong cold-stopping properties. Various attributes that'll help you fend off disease. Three of these are onions, garlic, and ginger as they have strong anti-viral and anti-bacterial properties. Anytime you start to feel a cold coming on eat a green onion, a large clove of garlic (not too be confused with a whole bulb), and about the same size of ginger all raw. It is powerful stuff and when you first try it, you may have difficulty getting it down. Try biting small bits at a time rather than the whole thing at once. But if you do this you may shorten the cold or even stop it in its tracks. That being said, if you eat these foods on a regular basis you may never have to worry about a cold coming on.

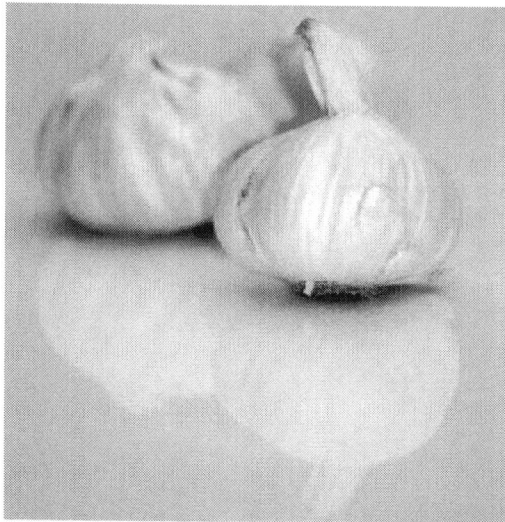

27
Super Foods

Not all foods are created equal. Not by a long shot. Some foods have way more nutrition in them. Compare a piece of white bread to raw cacao (chocolate in its natural form). The white bread has empty carbohydrates and possibly a few minerals from being enriched. The cacao has among the highest degree of antioxidants in the world. It is loaded with good fats, minerals, vitamins as well as phytonutrients not found in most foods. In fact, cacao is one of the most chemically complex of all foods out there. To go into different superfoods is beyond the scope of this book. Just realize there are foods out there that have way more bang for their buck like certain berries, algae, roots, fruits, seeds and more. Do you own research and start consuming them on a regular basis. Many can be found in local health stores these day but you can also find them online. Check out www.legendarystrength.com/go/superfoods

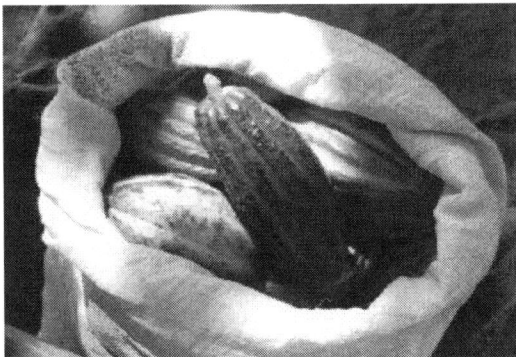

28
Adaptogenic Herbs

Just as certain foods have more quality nutrition in them than others, certain herbs are the same way. In Chinese medicine there is a class of herbs called the Superior herbs. These include Reishi, Ginseng, Cordyceps, Deer Antler, Ho Shou Wu and many others. These superior herbs are better in many ways, one of which is the ability to take them for long periods of time and only get good results due to their double direction activity. This is as opposed to inferior herbs which are only for certain times and certain ailments. Once again this is beyond the scope of this book. Do more research then start taking these wonderful herbs. I highly recommend the book <u>Radiant Health: The Ancient Wisdom of the Chinese Tonic Herbs</u> by Ron Teeguarden. My favorite formulas come from <u>www.legendarystrength.com/go/superiorherbs</u>

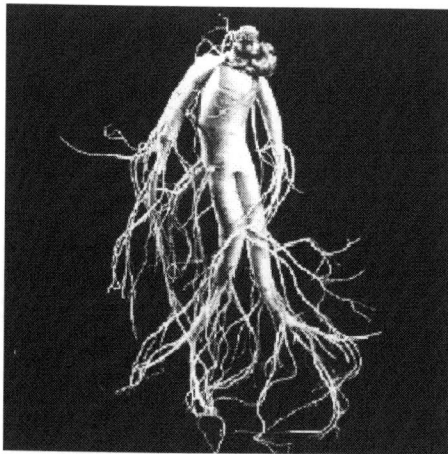

29
Mineralization

Minerals are very important. In fact, it could be said that mineralization equals health. Different minerals are used for all the functions of the body. And the majority of the population is deficient in many minerals. Some notable ones include magnesium and zinc. Due to our food being grown or raised in low quality conditions the minerals in most food, even organic, are on a downward trend and have been for many years. And don't think a cheap multivitamin will help you. In those, the minerals are in forms not readily available to your body. By eating quality foods, raw foods including many superfoods, as well as smart supplementation you can get all the minerals you need. Its something to think about because you most likely are deficient too. The minerals I've been using with great results are available from www.legendarystrength.com/go/minerals

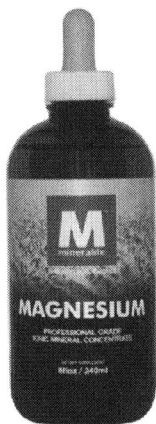

30
<u>*Do Away With Drugs*</u>

I'm not talking about recreational drugs, though that is something you should do without as well. I'm talking about pharmaceuticals. The problem with these drugs is that they treat symptoms not the root cause of issues. I realize in some cases, in certain treatments, they may have benefits but over the long haul you certainly shouldn't be on anything for life. And for small problems you shouldn't immediately reach for drugs. When you restore health in all these other areas of your life by following the tips in this book you should be able to cut down or out on what you take. I am not recommending you stop whatever you're on immediately but with proper medical supervision as your health improves you may be able to eventually do so.

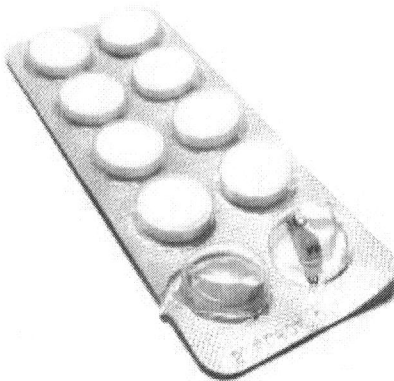

31
Fast For 24 Hours Once A Week

The body needs rest. This includes the digestive system which is highly energy intensive. Most people eat, eat and eat some more never giving the body time when its not processing food except in sleep. Even before the last meal is processed the next one starts. One habit that is a good thing to start is fasting for 24 hours once a week or once every other week. This period frees up energy that is normally used in processing food to be used for other important tasks like healing the body. Twenty-four hours is really not a long time to go, nor is it bad for the body in any way (unless diabetic or related issues). You can't go hungry in that time, even if you feel like you would. Plus it is great for developing will power, and lessening your reliance or even addiction to food.

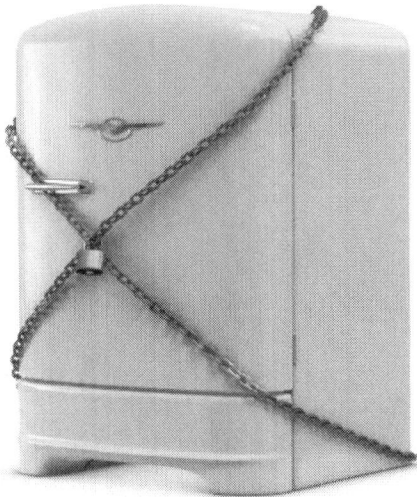

32
Fasting When Ill

Humans are the only animal that eats when sick. All others creatures stop eating. If your energy is being spent on digesting food then that is taking away from energy that can be used fighting the cold or disease. There are certain times when you want to eat. By becoming more in tune with your body you'll know the right time to break the fast. But by fasting anytime you begin to feel ill you can have it fully pass in 24-48 hours instead of it lasting for days or weeks. Even if you don't do a strict water fast look at eating foods that are more nutritious and easily digestible rather than large heavy cooked meals.

33
Longer Fasts

Fasting really is an art and a science. There are different ways to do it, drinking only water, drinking juices, liquid fasts, even eating fruits and vegetables. You can also go for much longer periods. Depending on how your health is, you could stand to gain from doing a 3-day or 1-week cleansing fast. If this seems like something you may be interested in I recommend you read Paul Bragg's book called <u>The Miracle of Fasting</u>.

34
Friction Bathing

The skin is the largest elimination organ in the body. More so then breathing. Thus, it stands to reason that you should keep it opened up. Unnatural lotions and makeups should be avoided, but you also must clear off the dead skin that accumulates. The best way to do this is with a brush or a rough towel. Scrub your body down as if you were drying yourself off after a bath, although its good to go over each area more than once. This can help to remove excess dead skin and should make it smoother and healthier.

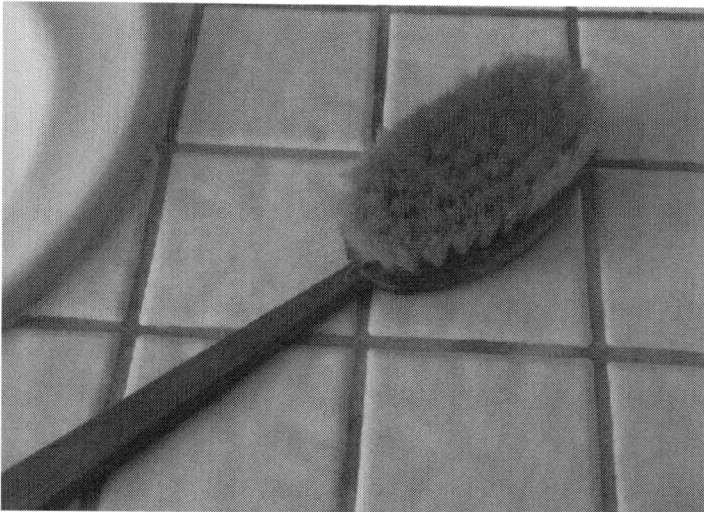

35
Shower Filter

Your drinking water isn't the only place you should have a higher quality water. If you take a hot shower the heat causes all the pores to open up in your body. Then the gases from what's in that water, like chlorine or fluorine, can easily get inside your body. In fact, the amount you get is far worse then what you would drink. A simple shower filter can be bought and easily attached to the head making your shower water instantly better. Not only will this improve your health but your skin and hair will end up smoother and softer.

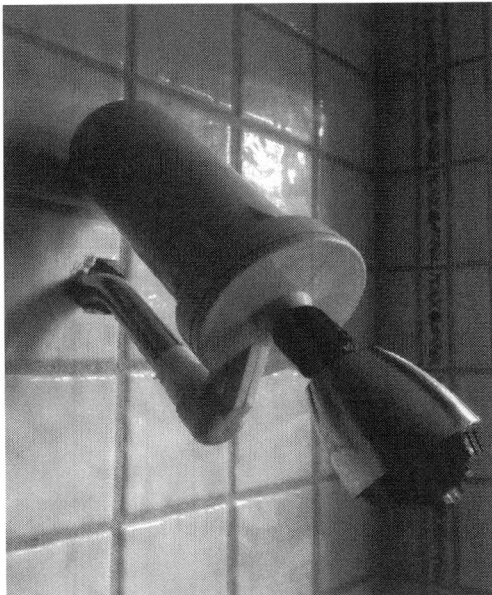

36
Cold Water Treatment

You ever jump into a cold pool or lake? Feel that rush of energy? This is actually very good for you to do. The shock of cold awakens the nerve force in the body. Some people, like the Polar Bear Club, even go so far as to work up to the ability to stay in freezing waters for prolonged periods of time. This increases your bodies ability to withstand not just the elements but much else. Now you don't want to start by jumping into freezing waters. Instead try turning your shower as cold as you can take it at least for a little bit of time. The worse this idea sounds to you, the more you likely need it.

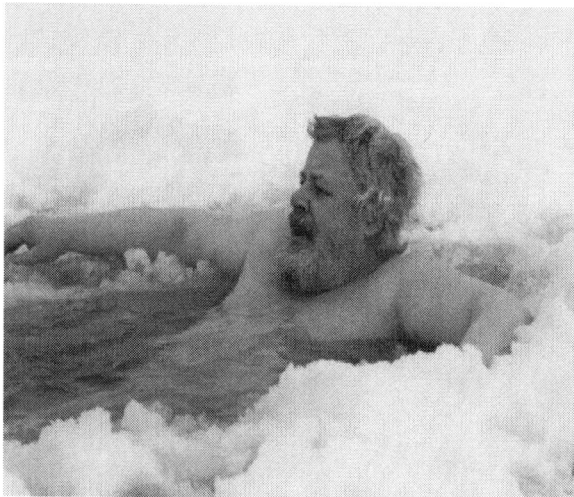

37
Hot Water Treatment

Hot water is also good for you. It helps you to relax. And relaxation is a good thing. After a tough day or hard training, soaking in a hot tub, or just taking a hot shower can feel great and recharge your body. Don't overdo it though or you'll end up feeling a bit sluggish.

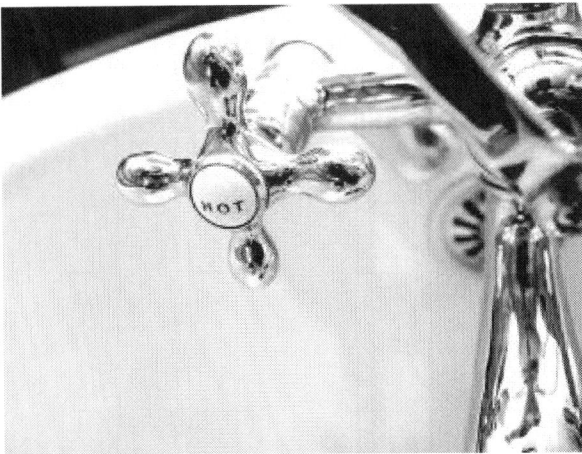

38
Alternating Cold And Hot

By contrasting the two different temperatures you'll get both the benefits and more. Blood is drawn to the skin in hot water and away in cold water. By going from one extreme to another you'll shock your body into action. I've heard its been called a Finnish Sauna, to go from a sauna then roll around in the snow and repeat. I've haven't personally done this one but would love to try it. As a kid I remember running from the hot tub to the pool back and forth many times. If you don't have anything else you can always use your shower to awaken your body and improve circulation.

39
Raise Feet When Using The Bathroom

Did you know that sitting down is actually just about the worst position to use the bathroom in as far as the design of our bodies is concerned? A much better position is to go into a full squat. As most people aren't going to do away with the toilet, myself included, the next best thing is to raise up your feet. Little stools (no pun intended) can be used or any sturdy object of low height. Alternatively you can raise up onto the balls of your feet if you have nothing else. This will aid in evacuation.

40
Poop Often

How many times per day do you eat? How many times per day do you evacuate your bowels? Those numbers should be close to the same. And anything less than once a day means your digestion and health isn't what it should be. This doesn't mean you need to take laxatives, just something you should be aware of, and will come to see as you improve your diet and health. Work with increasing the amount of fiber you take in, especially leafy vegetables, and you'll see this number go up. If you need a real boost in fiber try psyllium husk powder. Also avoid white flour. Back in the early 1900's white bread was prescribed as a surefire method of slowing up the colon. This and dairy can act essentially like glue in your system.

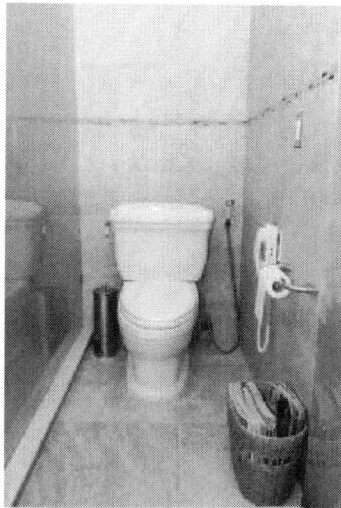

41
Brush And Floss

Most people brush their teeth. But take a look at what tooth paste you're using. Is it natural or is there big warnings not to swallow it? Should you be putting anything in your mouth you wouldn't swallow? Besides regularly doing this you need to floss. Flossing may be even more important to remove any food particles stuck between your teeth. Do these on a regular basis, along with a good diet and you'll never have any issues when you see the dentist.

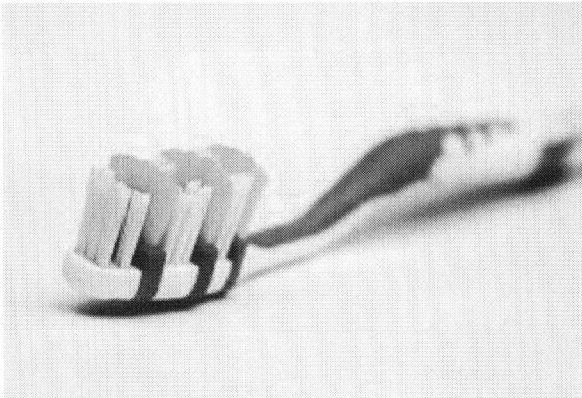

42
Tongue Scraping

The mouth is the most bacteria filled area in your body. The tongue holds much of it. You may brush and floss your teeth but do you ever clean your tongue? You should. Get a tongue scraper or an even better tool called the Ora-brush available at www.legendarystrength.com/go/orabrush, which utilizes bristles making tongue scraping even more effective. Besides keeping your mouth healthier as a side benefit you'll enjoy fresher breath.

43
Get More Sleep

This is another one I'm sure you already know. Your body and mind needs sleep. The more of it the better up to a certain point. But that point isn't even clear. Olympic athletes were studied with different groups getting different amounts of sleep. The group that slept twelve hours a day recovered best. Twelve hours may be out of the reach or desire of most of us. But you should at a bare minimum get seven hours of sleep every night. I go for an average of nine. If you aren't getting enough sleep think about how you can rearrange your life in order to get more. There are those that can get by on less but I would be careful of going too far.

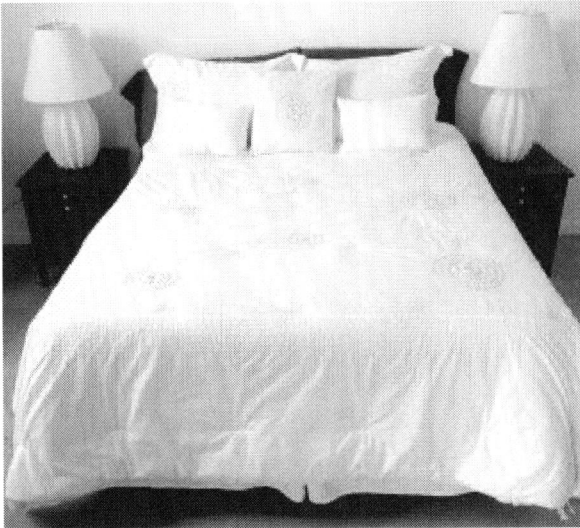

44
Make Up On Sleep

Life gets in the way of sleep sometimes. That's alright. A sign of a healthy person is someone who can go a night without sleep and still be alert and functional the following day. Suppose for several days you aren't able to get the quantity or quality of sleep you are use to. Make up for it. When you have the opportunity the best thing you can do to really recharge is sleep for 10 or 12 hours. This doesn't make up for a regular bad sleeping cycle but it can give you a boost to recovery.

45
Nap Time

Another way to fit in a little extra sleep is to take a nap midday. The circadian rhythm proves that this is a good idea in following with the body's cycle each day. Sometime between noon and 4 take a short 15-30 minute nap. Don't sleep longer as then you'll go into deep sleep and wake up groggy. And if you take a nap too late in the day it can mess with you falling asleep at night. Just this short time to 'go out' and you'll wake up refreshed and ready to go. This can also be great for boosting your recovery.

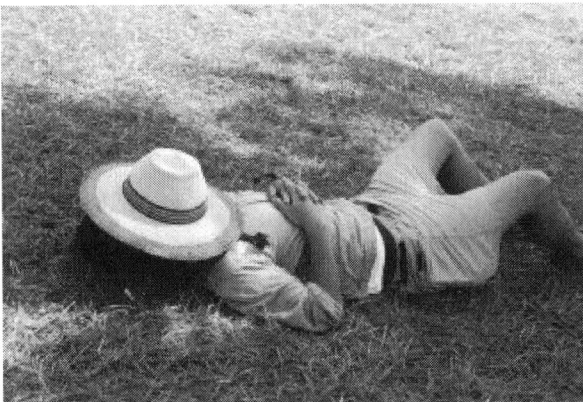

46
Improve The Quality Of Sleep

You need a certain quantity of sleep but of utmost importance is the quality of your sleep as well. By practicing many of the other guidelines in this book you should automatically start to sleep better. Better nutrition, not eating right before bed, cutting out or down on caffeine, eliminating noise and light are all easy steps. Another one is to think and believe you'll be getting a good night's sleep versus believing you'll wake up tired. If necessary you can look at natural sleep aids like melatonin that may aid you in getting a restful night's sleep.

47
Avoid Pillows

Pillows are not all they're cracked up to be. I remember first reading about this and thinking it was silly, but the truth is you only enjoy and need to sleep with a pillow because you've become accustomed to it. Just try this as an experiment and eliminate your use of pillows for a week especially if you sleep on your back. A small pillow if you sleep on your sides is alright but avoid too much cushioning as it puts your head in an unnatural position. With a raised head you're telling your body to be awake and at attention which kicks off hormones like adrenaline. Even better is to use the pillow to raise your feet rather then your head, putting yourself in a slightly inverted position.

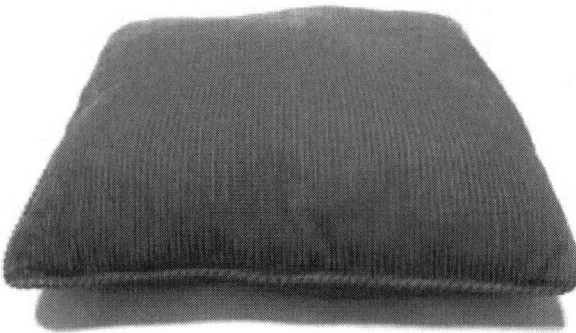

48
<u>Sleep On Your Back Or Sides</u>

The optimal way to sleep is on your back. It allows your body to work in the best manner and allow for the best breathing. Sleeping on the sides is a close second and many people find sleeping on the back difficult to do. What you want to avoid is sleeping on your stomach. This constricts breathing and should be avoided. It may take some time to adjust to a change but it can be done and will likely improve your quality of sleep.

49

Best Hours To Sleep

Big surprise here. You're suppose to sleep when the sun is down and get up when the sun does. This is the natural rhythm of things. Light regulates certain hormones, namely melatonin which is needed for quality sleep. Studies are beginning to find that those people which do not follow this, such as those who work night shifts, have more health problems than those who don't. And when the night gets longer? Maybe you should be sleeping longer in that season too. Regardless of this though, the best thing you can do is have regular hours. This way your body becomes accustomed to doing the same thing every day at the same time. When it doesn't have to guess what's going on it'll be more efficient.

50
Take Pulse In Morning

You can do this in order to become more in tune with what your body tells you. The first thing you do when you wake up in the morning is note your pulse rate. In general a lower pulse means you're healthier. If you notice your pulse is higher than normal, whether this is stress from work, or doing too much in the gym, you'll want to ease back until your pulse returns to normal. In order to be effective you'll want a timer right next to your bed so you don't have to get up to do it as that would increase your pulse rate immediately.

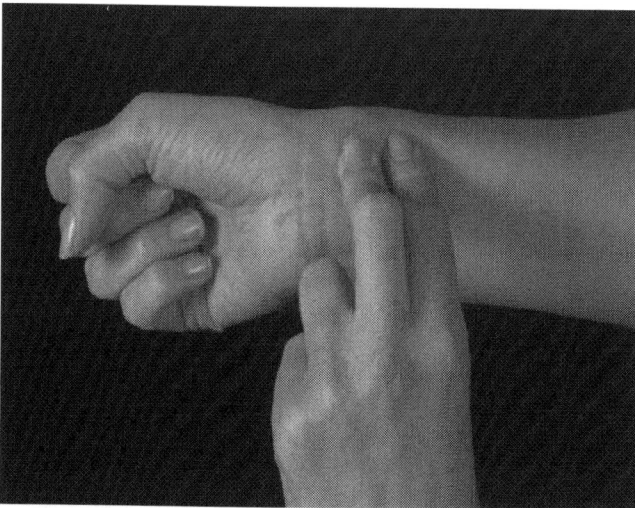

51
Joint Mobility

How well can you move? Do you have the ability to move each joint in a full range of motion as it should be able to move? If not you should work on it. From what I've seen the worse areas for the majority of people are the pelvis and spine (the lumbar, thoracic, and cervical areas). Of course, if you've had past injuries you may have different problems areas. Lack of movement is dis-use, which overtimes makes it so that you can't move those areas. So move those joints and keep them healthy.

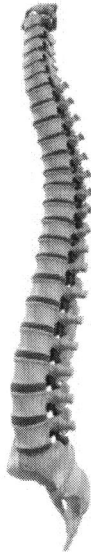

52
Strength Training

Strength training is not just for athletes and bodybuilders. Everyone can and should be doing it. Why? Properly done progressive strength training builds muscle, bone density and helps to optimize the hormones. It creates density and stability where it is needed in the body. You can do it in many ways, lifting weight, bodyweight exercises, kettlebells and much more. There is too much about training to get into here. Find a basic program and stick to it. For more information on this and the following tips check out www.legendarystrength.com

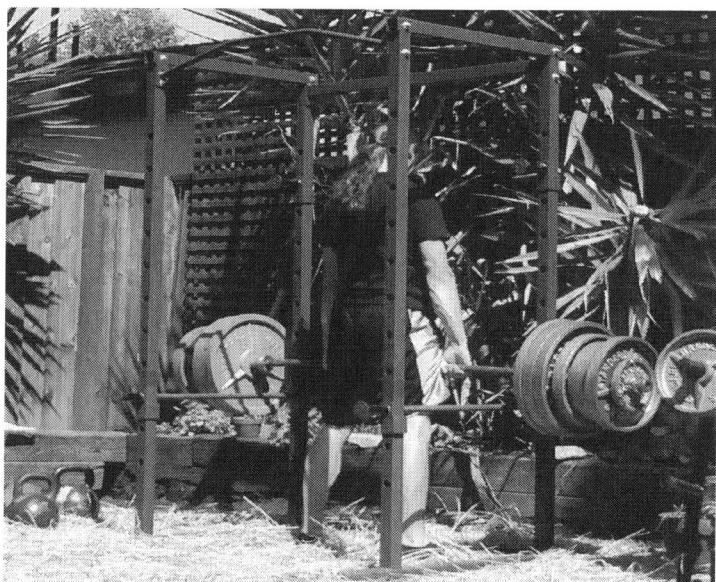

53
Conditioning

The flip side of strength training is conditioning. Are you able to run a mile without being completely spent afterward? Even if you can lift large weights, but get winded by climbing a flight of stairs you are not in shape. The heart and lungs need to be built up as well as the rest of the body. Once again there are many ways you can go about this. Even strength training done in a circuit fashion can work to build your conditioning so that it takes no extra time.

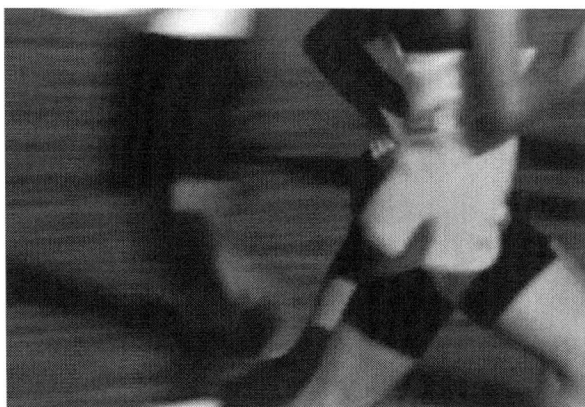

54
Train Your Entire Body

Does any part of your body deserve strength and health less than any other? No. Therefore, you should train your entire body. Some of the common areas neglected by most are the hands, neck and feet. You don't need to train each muscle individually with isolation exercises. Instead pick the big compound exercises that work more of the body all at once. If, when you look at your program, you're missing anything add it in. This helps to make sure you have no weak links.

55
Build Flexibility

You need enough flexibility to get through your daily life plus a little extra. For most people this isn't much. I would add you should be capable of easily, without strain, squatting all the way down and staying there comfortably, bending over and touching the floor, and locking both arms out overhead. If you do not have this flexibility work within your limits over time to build it. This can go along with your mobility work and even strength training, depending on how you do it.

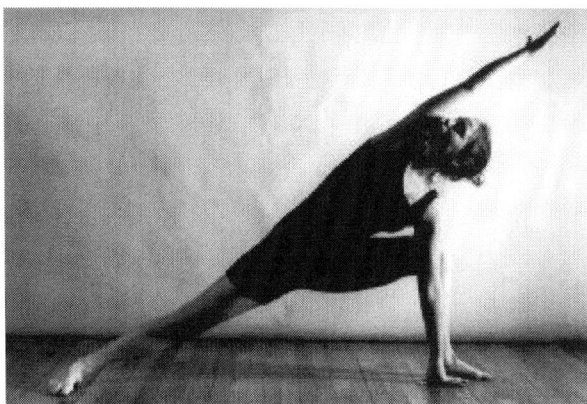

56
Choose Anaerobic Over Aerobic

Anaerobic exercise is exercise done without oxygen. It refers to the process your body goes through to produce energy. Aerobic exercise is done with oxygen. As an example, sprinting is anaerobic while jogging is aerobic. Studies are showing anaerobic exercise is more important and that it transfers over to aerobic but not vice versa. So instead of running for miles and constantly trying to do more you should do intervals, sprinting then jogging, repeated back and forth. Personally I prefer hill sprints. Besides running you have many other options including kettlebell swings or snatches, club swinging, rowing and more.

57
Natural Movements

Certain exercises are better than others. Doing a curl in a machine may help to build strength. But that strength is likely to only work in that locked-in, stable plane the machine creates. Going to free weights is a step in the right direction. Going towards more natural movements is even better. What are natural movements? Watch a kid have fun in a playground. Running, jumping, rolling, falling, crawling on all fours, swinging from bars, climbing and the like are all something you'll see. Those are natural movements and those are all abilities you and your body should be capable of regardless of your age.

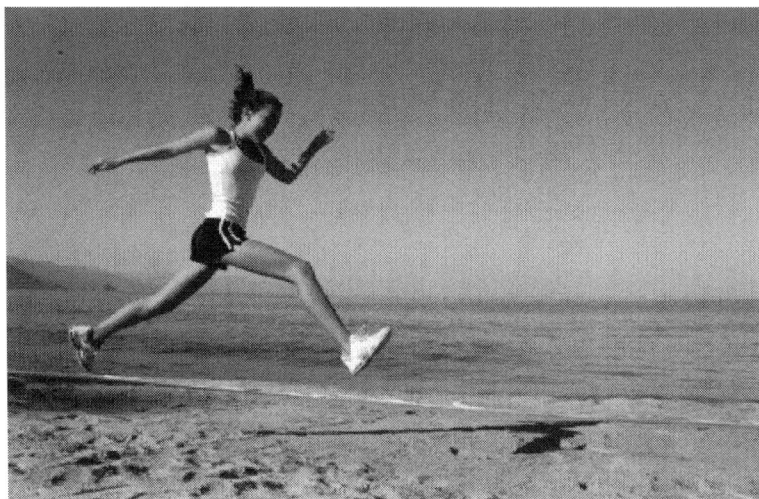

58
Abdominal Vacuum

Want to massage your organs? Squeeze them to make sure they're working? Do the abdominal vacuum. This is great for your organs, elimination and it can be fun to do. Bend over and blow all your air out. Raise your diaphragm thereby creating a vacuum in your stomach. This makes your waist seem very small when compared to normal. With practice you'll be able to get a more pronounced look in the vacuum. A set of ten every morning is a good place to start and can be done with your breathing exercises. Make sure you do it on an empty stomach though.

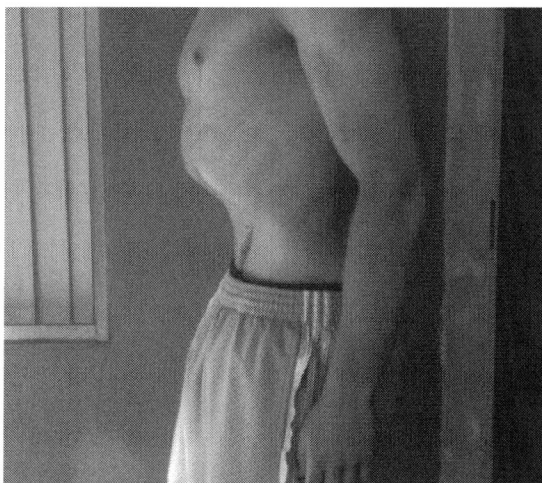

59
Hanging For Decompression

Your body must battle gravity all day long. But you can use gravity to your advantage too. Hang from something overhead, like a pullup bar or sturdy tree branch, and gravity will pull on your body to decompress your spine. Want even more? Use a yoga swing, gravity boots or something similar to hang upside down to decompress. This allows your spine to open up, which can balance it out from being pulled down all day.

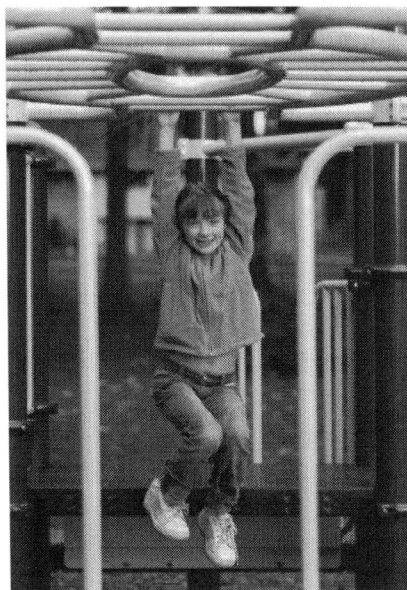

60
Maintain Good Posture

As was previously mentioned gravity weighs down on us all day, every day. We've all seen old people hunched over. This is the result of several things one of which is bad posture compounded overtime, plus a lack of flexibility and mobility. Simply remind yourself anytime you find yourself hunched over to sit or stand up straight. Good posture is largely a habitual thing. Besides that, effective strength training will help you with this issue.

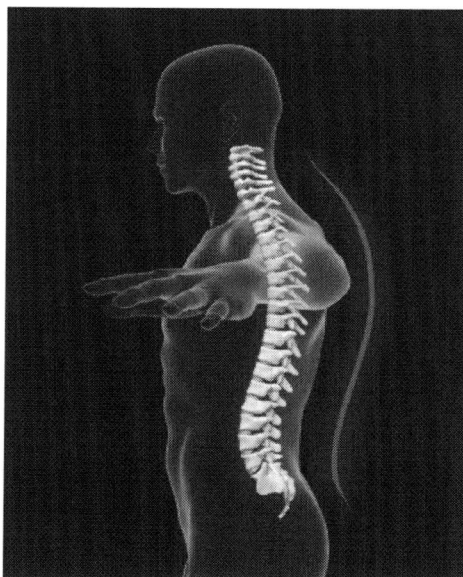

61

Inversion

Did you know almost all animals die with arthritis in their bones? That is except for two, bats and possums. Two creatures which sleep upside down. I'm not recommending you start sleeping inverted but for great health you should spend some time with your hips over your heart and your heart over your head. This reverses the flow of gravity and helps to remove stagnation found in the lower limbs. There are several methods of doing this. You can do a headstand or a handstand. You can also hang from a bar or attachment if you have gravity boots or some kind of swing setup to combine decompression with inversion. However you do it, if you can work up to half an hour a day of inversion you'll be healthier for it.

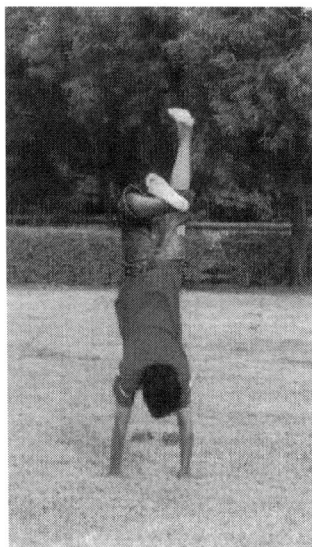

62
Sweat

Sweat is formed when the body is trying to cool itself down due to an increase in external and/or internal temperature. The skin is the largest organ system in the body and it needs to purge toxins and other waste products. Getting a sweat on is the way to do this. Vigorous exercises are the easiest way. Also if you have access to a sauna you're in luck. Anyway you can do it, regularly sweating, at least a few times each week, is great for your health.

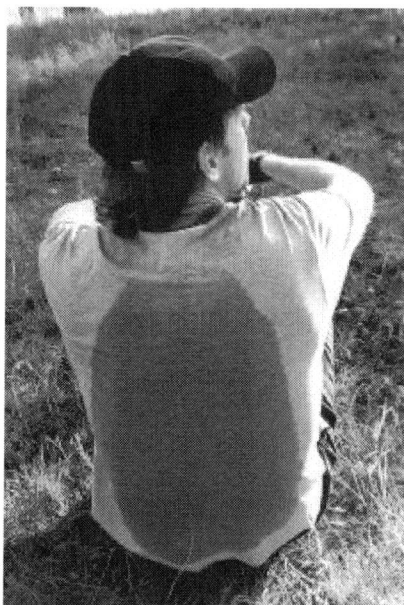

63
Walk On All Fours

While we may have evolved to walk upright it does come at it's costs. Walking and running on all fours is not only good exercise but inverts the body as well. This is commonly called a bear crawl and can be done forwards, backwards and to the sides. It is one of those natural movements discussed earlier. Try it out and you'll see what it can do for you. As one old health book I read stated, if you have time for one exercise, this may be it.

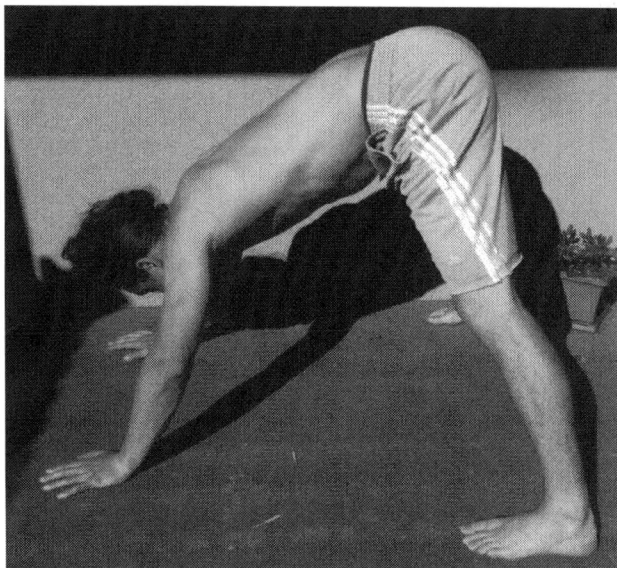

64
Energy Work

Your energy can be manipulated and this is a skill like anything else. By practicing some form of energy work you can make sure your energetic body is working as well as the physical one. If everything in the Universe is energy as quantum physics is showing us, restoring and maintaining a healthy energy body will do wonders for the physical body. Start practicing some form of Qi Gong, Tai Chi, or a similar method. For an in-depth resource on manipulating your own energy and even others, check out Energy Work by Robert Bruce.

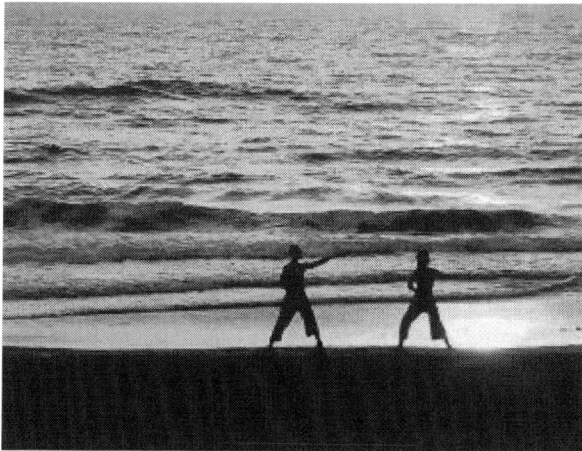

65
Bodywork

Bodywork of many types does more than just feel good. It can help restore the body to its natural functions. Certain areas of stagnation can be manipulated and broken up to allow the blood to flow through with massage. Other modalities can realign the body into its proper state. Find a skilled practitioner and then get regular bodywork done. Though nothing comes close to a skilled expert, if you're on a budget try swapping with a partner or some self massage.

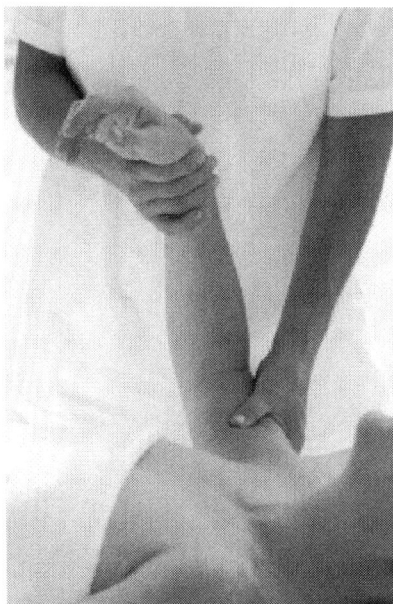

66
Reflexology/Acupuncture

According to Chinese medicine there are point on the hands, feet and even ears that correspond to every other area of the body. In addition there are energetic pathways that run up and down the body. Skilled practitioners can identify and help problems in any area of your body by manipulating these energy pathways. As before in bodywork, you may want to seek out an expert and get some work done. There are also ways you can tap into these areas yourself if you know what to do.

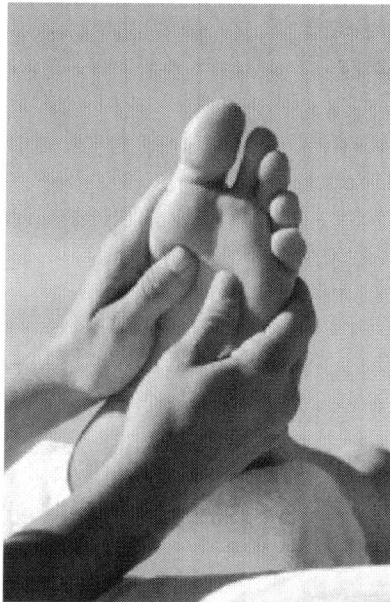

67
Walking After Dinner

After you eat dinner it's a good time to go for a nice leisurely stroll. As dinner is often the heaviest meal of the day this motion can aid in digestion and help you to relax. This can be combined with meditation, visualization, deep breathing or just having a good time conversing with others. It's the perfect way to unwind from the events of the day. Keep the pace slow as this is not an effort to get anywhere.

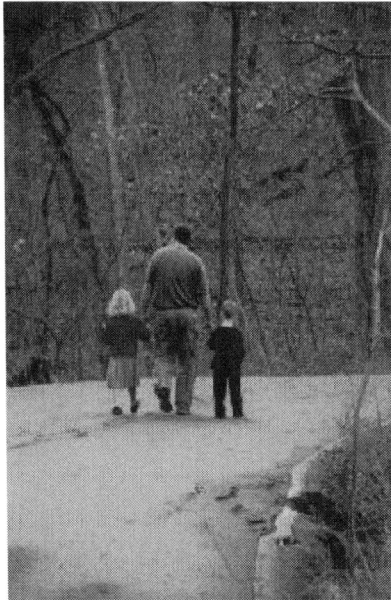

68
Go Barefoot

Shoes may be one of the worst inventions ever. As time goes on and they add more engineering to the shoes the worse it gets. The foot's natural architecture is, big surprise here, best and doesn't need improvement. Shoes close in the toes together (with some being much worse than others). Thick heeled running shoes change the way we run and then we wonder why we get knee or back pain. Well, you're not suppose to strike the ground with your heel on each step. Try that barefoot and you'll see that you're suppose to run on the ball of your foot. Ditch the shoes at least as much as you can. Or get a pair of more natural shoes that allow your feet to work as they're suppose to.

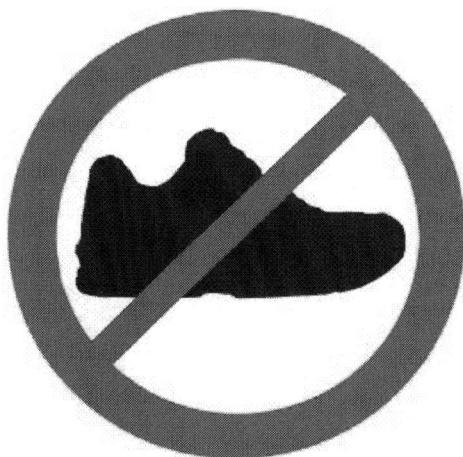

69
Connection with the Earth

Another issue with shoes is the rubber. This insulates us from the earth. So does being inside in our buildings. For optimal health you want to maintain a connection to the earth as much as possible. Studies show that this improves blood circulation, eases inflammation, increases quality of sleep, decreases muscle soreness, offers protection from harmful electric fields and much more. Try to spend at least half an hour a day in connection with the earth. If this is hard to do with your lifestyle, or you want more, they have technologies available that allow you to be grounded in your home and even bed. As I write this in my home office I am grounded via a pad at my feet. Find out more on the research as well as the technology at www.legendarystrength.com/go/earthing

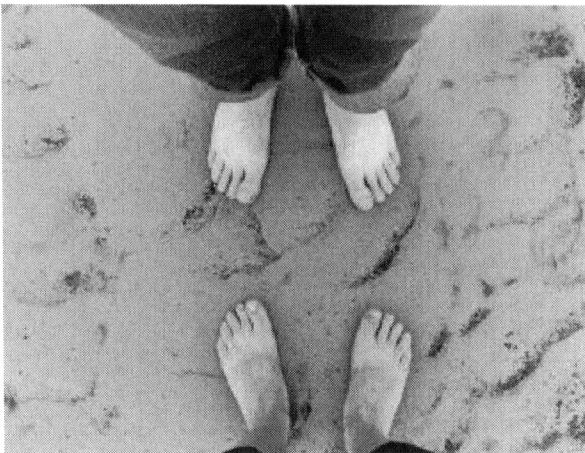

70
Get Outside In Nature

It can be hard to always be indoors or in cities. Besides the earth connection it just feels good to get outdoors in nature. I'm all for the amenities of modern life but you can't do away with Mother Nature completely. If you need to go camping, hiking, or take a trip to the beach that is fine. Get out there and get in touch. Plan a trip right now. Get your hands dirty. And have fun doing it.

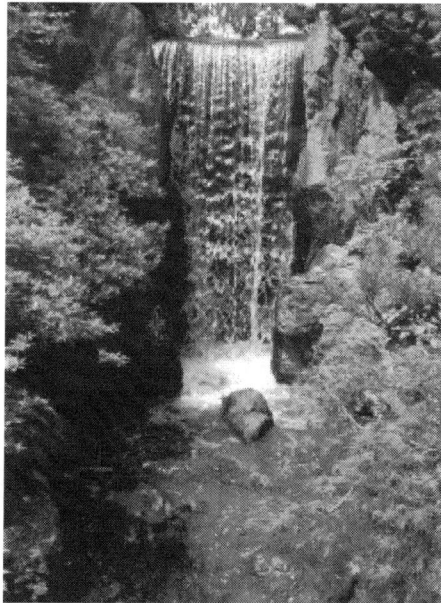

71
Get Sunlight

Sunlight is good for you in moderation. Not only does it produce Vitamin D (a necessary vitamin, one that many people are deficient in and may need to supplement orally). But when it contacts your skin it can produce good feelings. I know for myself, its much easier to get down in the cloudy and rainy winter months. You need the direct contact so avoid sunscreens, especially those with harsh chemicals in them. Get only enough sun as your body can handle and no more. Over time you'll be able to increase this amount.

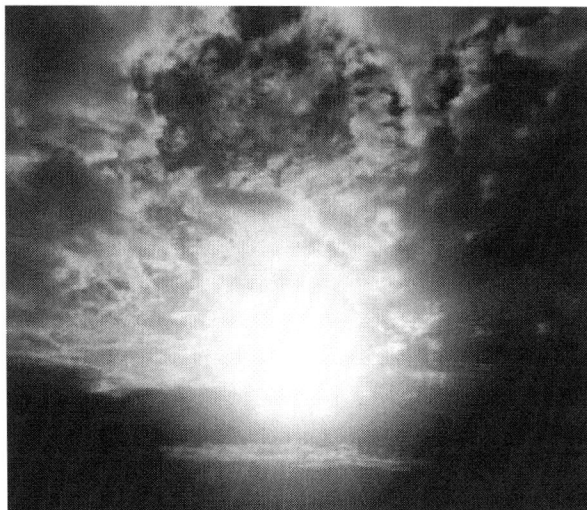

72
Sun Gazing

Sunlight is good for you, not just on your body (of course in moderation) but also for your eyes. There is an ancient Yogic practice called sun gazing which is the act of staring at the sun. You only want to do this for the first couple minutes when the sun comes up or the first couple minutes when the sun goes down. The angle of the sun in relation to the atmosphere makes this a healthful practice rather than burning out your eyes which it would do at most other times (and is not recommended). Some say that this practice can enhance your eyesight and provide you with direct energy from the sun. I'll leave you to further research and experiment yourself and see what you find. For best results make sure you're grounded when sun gazing.

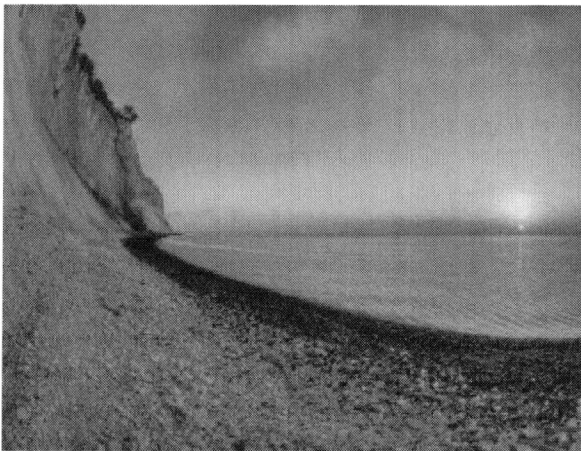

73
Meditate

Meditation is the act of focusing on one thing in order to quiet the mind. This can be breath counting, chanting a mantra, or staring at a mandala or candle flame. Properly done meditation synchronizes the hemispheres of the brain and takes you from beta brain waves to alpha and even lower, as it quiets the mind. I don't know about you but I always found meditation hard to do. Enter technology that makes it easy and even more effective. I highly recommend you check out Holosync from www.legendarystrength.com/go/holosync

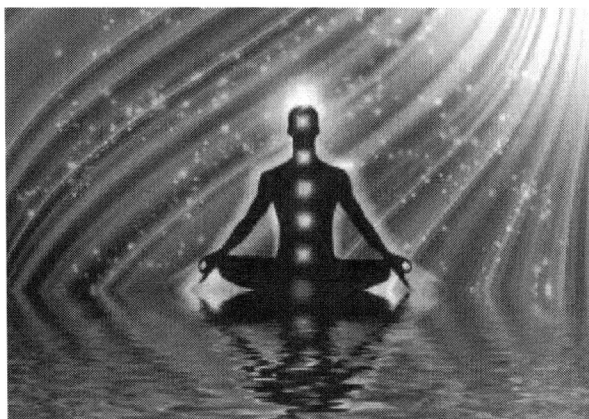

74

EMF Protection

Electromagnetic frequencies come in a wide variety. Some are bad for our body. Some are good. Those emitted from most household electronics and cell phones are in the bad category. If you doubt this you can try a simple test. Put you head up to a live TV for several minutes and see if you feel any difference. These EMF's can disrupt the natural ways our bodies' function. There are many books and articles online that go into depth on this subject. There are also many devices that can offer protection, though it's hard to say what really works and what doesn't. The simplest way is to get grounded with the earth as was described earlier.

75
Magnetism

The earth use to have a much stronger magnetic force to it. But over time this has dwindled to about one tenth what it use to be. Introducing strong magnetism back into our lives may be a good thing. There are certain areas in the earth that have stronger magnetic fields. But if you can't find one of those, various magnetic products, such as those found at www.legendarystrength.com/go/magnets are available which allow you to get the benefits of magnetic forces. You only want to use the north polarity of these magnets.

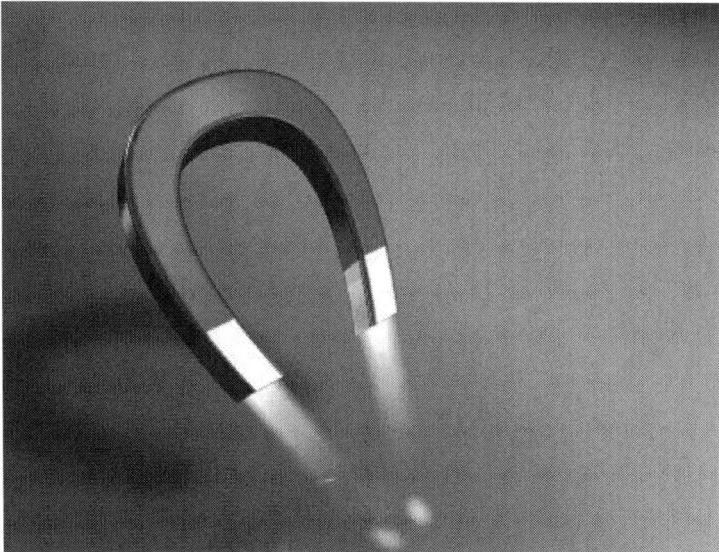

76
Test Hormone Levels

In order to be healthy you need optimal hormone levels. Proper diet and exercises will help to keep these levels in check. However, knowing is half the battle. There are relatively inexpensive saliva tests you can take at home and mail in to find out your hormone levels. Once you have these results you can manipulate what you do and eat in order to bring up any deficient levels.

77
Make More Money

If you want to be healthy you'll have to be able to afford more than 99 cent cheeseburgers. Many of the tips I've given you are free and can be done easily. Some only take a change in beliefs which can even be instant. But others may require some investment. Certain health technologies cost money, in addition to the regular buying of high quality food and supplements. I've heard it before and at times felt the same way, that organic food is expensive. But by increasing your income you'll be able to enjoy the better food without issue. Plus lack of money is a big cause of stress in most people's lives. Today more than ever, money is readily available for those that know how to acquire it.

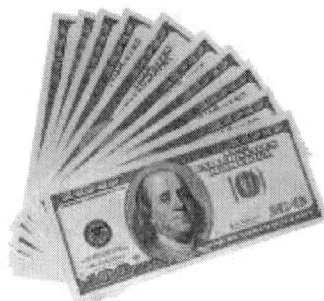

78
Choose Where You Live

You do have the choice. Hate the weather or the area? Then move! You can relocate to any area of the world you want to with some effort. If you enjoy the sun and heat move to a place where it stays sunny most of the time. Don't have access to fresh local food? Find a place that does. Your choices impact your happiness and health. This is a big one.

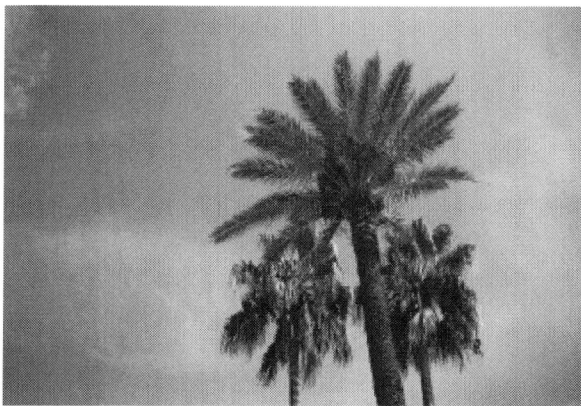

79
Cut Down On Or Out TV

TV is probably one of the biggest time wasters out there. If you looked at any of the previous points and said I don't have time for that, yet you spend hours in front of the tube each day, you need to look at your priorities. And when you're too tired to do anything when you come home from work besides plop down on the couch, realize you need to give energy first in order to get it back. Now I realize there are some good shows out there, and I'm a huge fan of movies. But instead of wasting hours of your day watching mindless programming, use a little as a reward for a day well spent. Not to mention the advertising and messaging coming through TV, especially the negative news, is anything but helping you attain health.

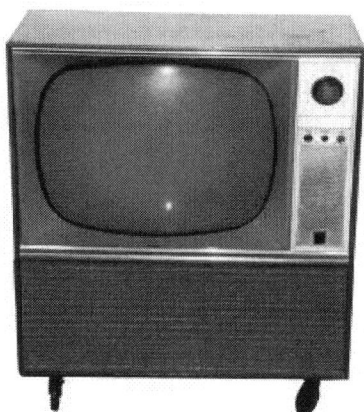

80
Be A Lifelong Learner

Use it or lose it. The same principle that works with your body works with your brain. If you want to maintain wit, intelligence and a good memory you must use these capabilities. The best way to keep the brain healthy is to continually add new connections by learning new things (in whatever you're interested in). There is so much information out there, literally at your fingertips via the internet. Learning about things you enjoy, not only will use your brain, but you'll find fulfillment from it.

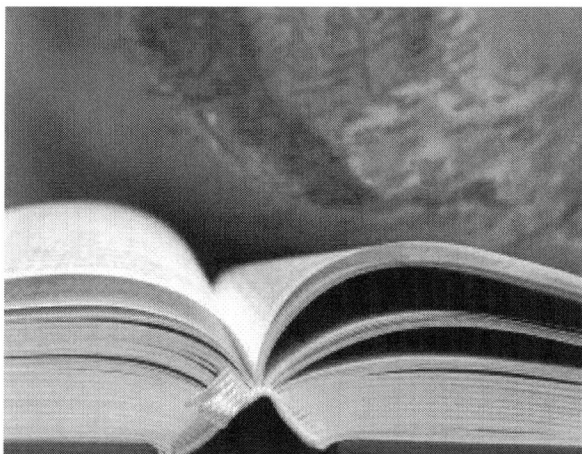

81
Work Right & Left Brain

I already mentioned using your brain, but are you using both sides? You need to. The left brain is highly logical, and most people in our society are trapped into only using this side. The right brain is artistic and creative. This can take many forms. Don't say that you aren't any good at it and give it up. Instead get started and you can improve your skills. Overtime you may surprise yourself. By doing so you'll further unlock your own genius. I recommend reading How to Think Like Leonardo Da Vinci by Michael Gelb for details and exercises on how to do this.

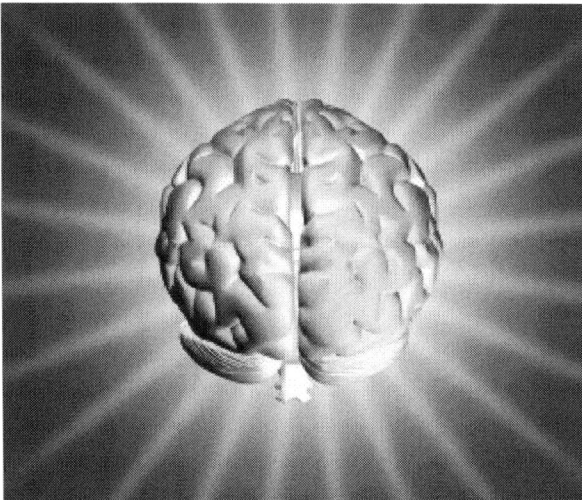

82
Mental Attitude

Do you think of yourself as a healthy person? Or do you think that you always have problems and get sick all the time? What you think and the beliefs you have about yourself do matter. If nothing else they'll help you to do the things that will actually improve your health. For some a simple switch can be made but these attitudes are largely unconscious. Using different techniques like hypnosis, NLP or EFT may be the shortcut you need. If necessary find a skilled practitioner in your area to help you.

83
Live Stress Free

Stress will bog down your immune system. You ever notice how your body will shut down after being stressed out for too long a time? Not all stress is bad but too much definitely is. Do the things that will help you do away with the stress in good ways. And one idea to live by is to let whatever happens be okay. The different ideas in the book should help you to raise your threshold of what stress effects you as well as deal with any stress you do have in healthy ways.

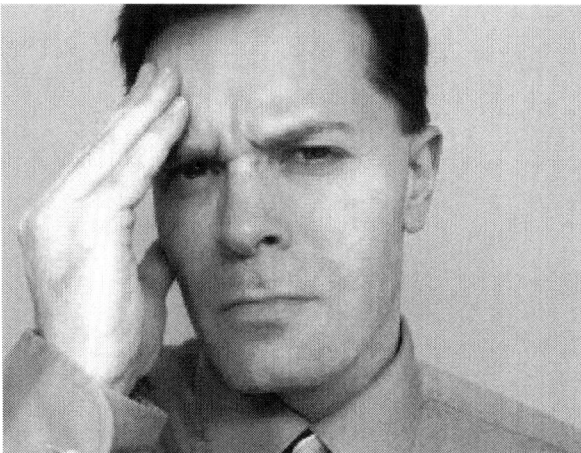

84
Invincibility Belief

Going back to beliefs from earlier. Why not take this to the extreme? What if you truly believed that you never got sick? Even if you do end up sick, are you going to think that tomorrow is going to be even worse, or do you go to bed thinking you'll be back to 100% the next morning. You may not be but you will get over it faster than someone who doesn't. At the same time cultivate a belief in invincibility. Go through life where nothing can hurt you. Obviously this is not something you want to put to the test. But what if it helps you get by without ever getting injured? If it does, you might as well use it.

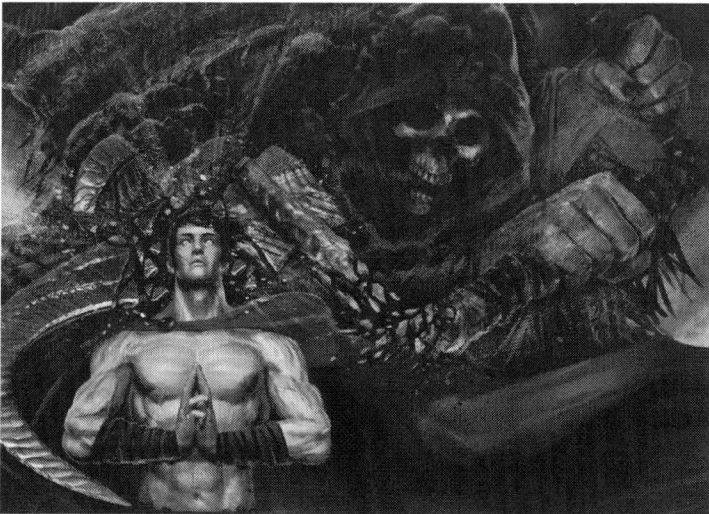

85
Don't Believe In Aging

Its not necessary to age. Sure the time you've been here on earth does increase with each year. But it isn't a downward slope to the end. We have the knowledge and technologies to stop and even reverse the symptoms and causes of what most people think is aging. The truth is time itself is not toxic. Its all the other things that happen over time. Do you think the last years of your life will be horrible, unable to recognize your friends or family and barely the ability to move? Do you think it all ends when your 70? Or do you think you will go on past 100 in great health. The choice is yours and it starts with belief.

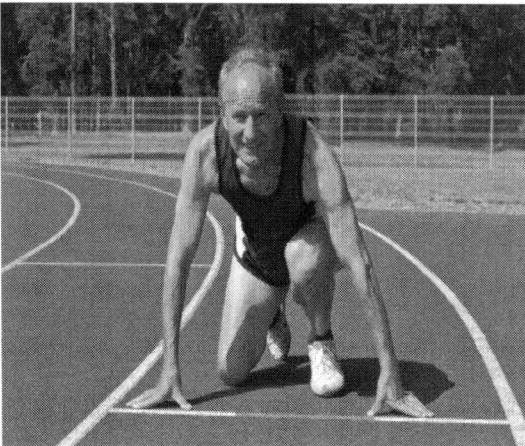

86
<u>*Decide To Be Healthy*</u>

Health first starts with a decision. If you make that decision everything else will start to come to be. But this must be a real decision. It can't be a wishy-washy idea that you'll ditch in a couple days or weeks. Once you make that decision, more information, better food and technologies will make themselves apparent to you. You have this book so you're already on the right track but this isn't the end. In fact, there is no end point, but a constant journey.

87
<u>Decide To Be Happy</u>

At the same time you can make a decision to be happy. Happiness is not really effected by your outside circumstances. It is really a choice. Surveys found that those in America and those in the third world tended to be just as happy as each other regardless of the economic differences. Choose to be happy and you will be happier than someone who doesn't make that choice. I'm not saying you'll never get down but overall you'll do much better.

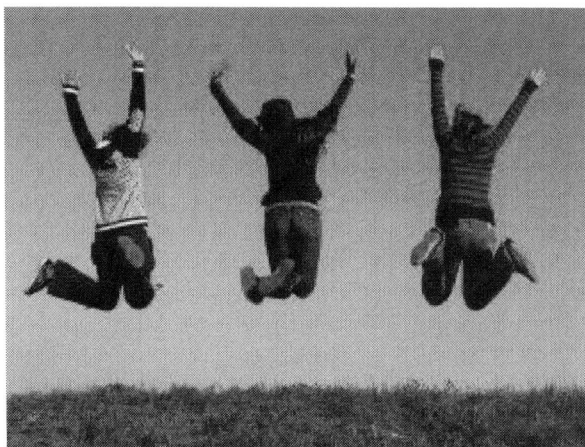

88
Picture Yourself Radiantly Healthy

How do you see and think of yourself? Go ahead and picture yourself in your mind right now. Do you see someone who always has health problems? Or do you see someone is is always healthy and has vigor? You make these mental pictures all the time whether you realize it or not. These mental pictures have a big impact on what comes to be. This image can easily be manipulated into a better image. I recommend you check out <u>Psycho-Cybernetics</u> by Dr. Maxwell Maltz for info on how to do this in the theater of your mind.

89
Do Something You Love

Happiness is a big part of health. If you lead a happy life you're likely to be healthier. We already know that happiness starts with a choice. On top of that a big part is doing something you love to do. Something that gives you fulfillment. Whatever that is find it and do it. It may take some time to get there but that time will pass whether you're working towards your dream or not, so you might as well start now. If you have no idea what that is at this time, start moving in the direction you think it might be. Where you start going seldom ends up exactly as you planned it anyway. But going in that direction opens up new doors. Having a mission in life will keep you healthier as you need that health in order to fulfill it.

90
Be Social

Humans are social creatures. It is a necessary thing to get out there and mix it up with people you do know and those you don't. Whether you're a natural at this or not doesn't matter. Of course, you should do those social activities that you enjoy. When you do that you'll be happier and thus healthier. Often when you are feeling down and trapped in your own mind this is the simple and easy cure. I'll leave you to find the right amount of socializing you need. Online activities do not make up for the real thing.

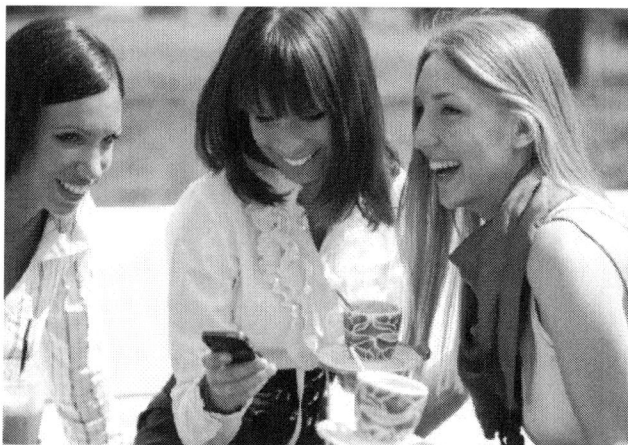

91
Avoid Unhealthy People

The people you associate with will impact you more than you know. They say look at your ten closest friends. If you average what they make financially you'll be right there in the middle. The same could be said for health. Do you get together with friends and talk about the latest injuries, illnesses, misery and death? If you do, you might want to look at what you're focusing on there. Get around healthy people and they'll bring you up rather than down.

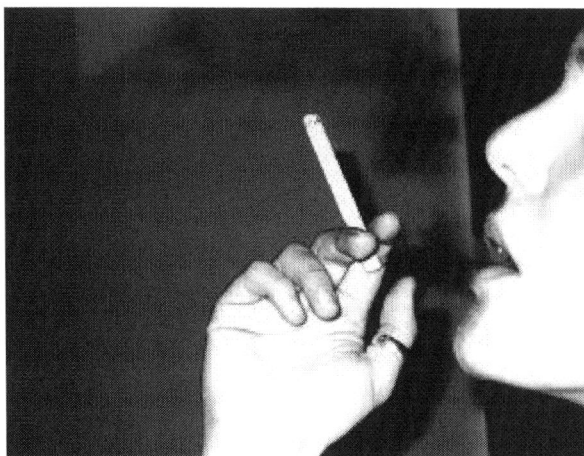

92
Laughter

I'm sure you have heard the statement that laughter is the best medicine. They even have what they call laughter yoga where people consciously work on laughing. I prefer getting around funny friends or watching good comedy. Laughing is fun to do and it helps to relax the body. Without a sense of humor you'll become an angry or sad person. Next time you're laughing just try not being happy and see how well it works.

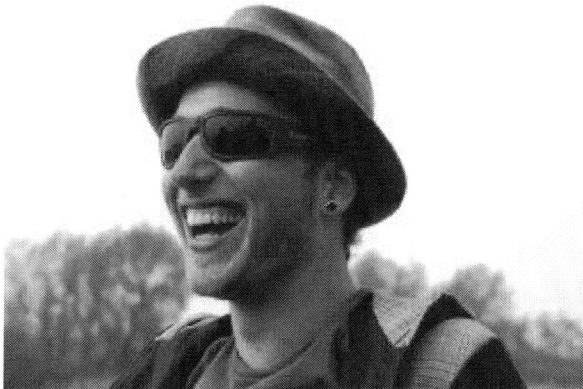

93
Smile

Want to be happy? Smile. It doesn't only work the other way. You can be happy and then smile or you can smile and then you'll be happy. Happiness leads to health. This is an easy one that you can start doing right now. An advanced tip is to smile on the inside as well as the out. Have an injury or problem? Direct that smiling, happy, fun energy into the area.

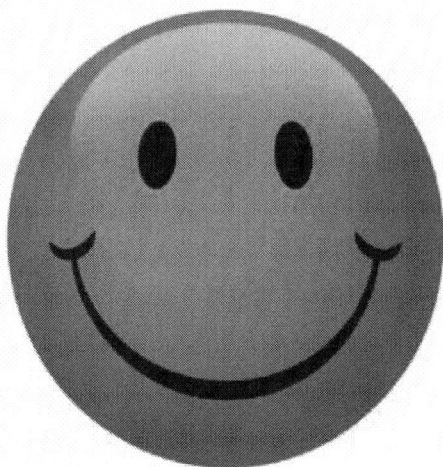

94
Play Games & Be Child Like

How happy are kids playing their games? Wouldn't you like to be more like that? Sure, as adults we have more responsibility but there needs to be times when you can just let go completely and get lost in the moment. If you have kids play with them. If you don't, find some fun, child-like activities you can engage in with your friends. If you need to, schedule the time so you can actually go out and do this. Playing, especially if its combined with physical activity, is great for your health. It brings laughter, fun, and good energy into your life.

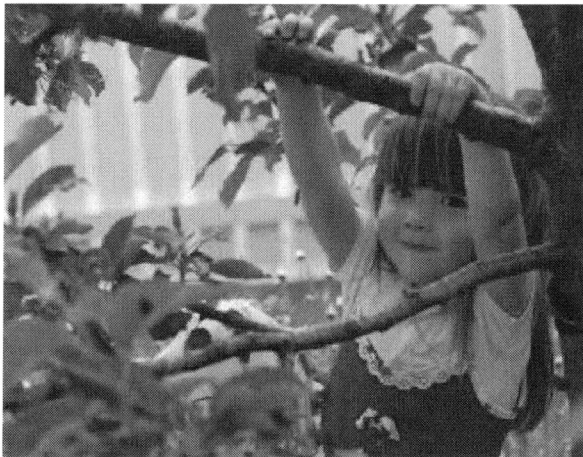

95
Good Sex Life

Humans are sexual creatures. After all that is how you were created. Though sex is responsible for much shame, anger, and other negativity a healthy sex life is good for you. Even necessary. Not only can it make you happy and establish closer bonds with your partner, but orgasm has been shown to release certain healthful hormones in the body, such as Oxytocin. As with anything this can be done too much, especially for men who lose something with every ejaculation.

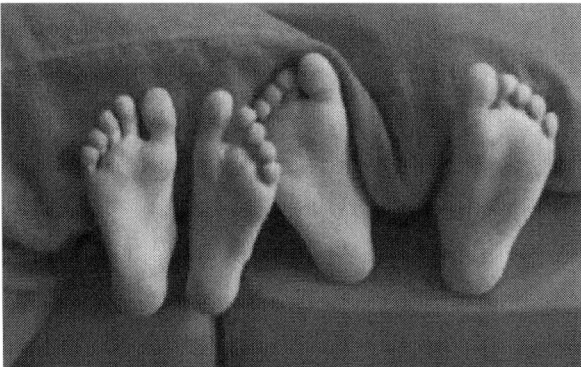

96
Converse With Eating

A great time to be social is when you're eating. One of the reasons this helps is that it tends to slow down our eating. This may seem to be in contrast to tip 13 but I believe its the one good exception. By slowing down and having to talk you'll be more in touch with your hunger than shoveling some food down by yourself before you move onto the next thing. It combines socializing with food bringing two good things together.

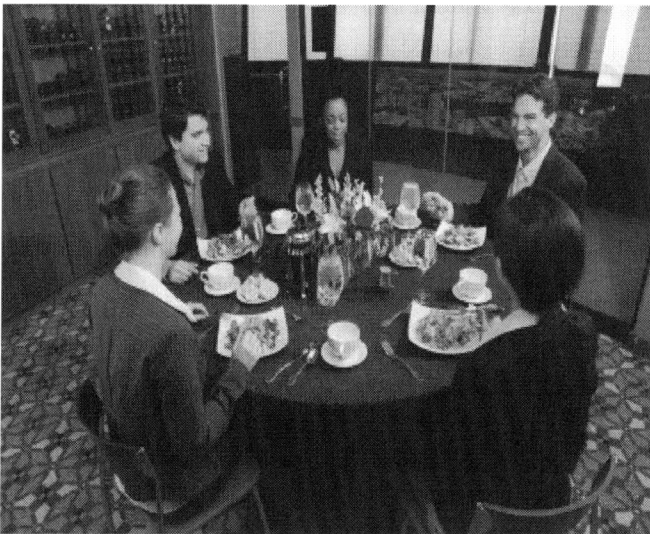

97
Don't Take Life Too Seriously

Life is a game. Have fun when you play it. This goes along with a sense of humor. When we get too wrapped up in our mind on the details we lose sight of the big picture. The big picture is to relax and have fun. After all in the grand scheme of things what does all that you do amount to, if you expand out thousands of years or outside of Earth? The healthiest and happiest people I've met do not take life too seriously.

98
Get A Health Partner

Going alone is seldom as fun as teaming up with a partner. If you can find a friend or loved one who can take this journey towards health with you all the better. Get together and talk about what you're doing. Compare results and experiences. Learn from each other in what each person is doing and what is working for them. You'll gain added insights and not feel like you're going it alone.

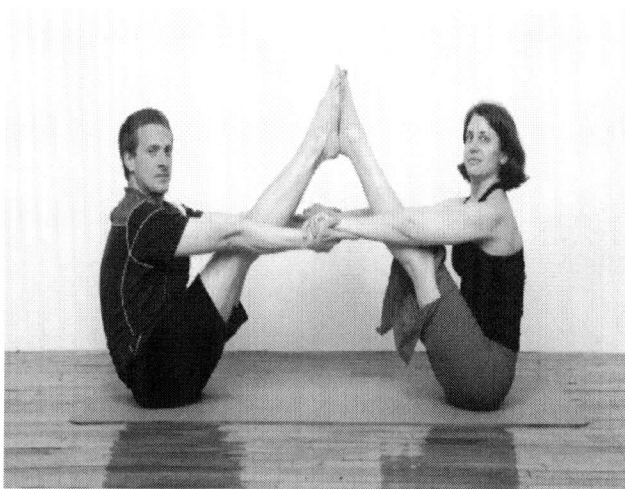

99

Love

Love is one of the most powerful emotions we have. It is positive and it feels good to be in love and to be loved. Enjoy it. This starts with loving yourself. If you do not truly do that any other love you give or receive will be a shallow shell of what it can be. Once that is complete seek out the right partner for yourself. Behind every great man is a great woman and vice versa. There are different forms of love, enjoy them all and you'll live a healthier and longer life.

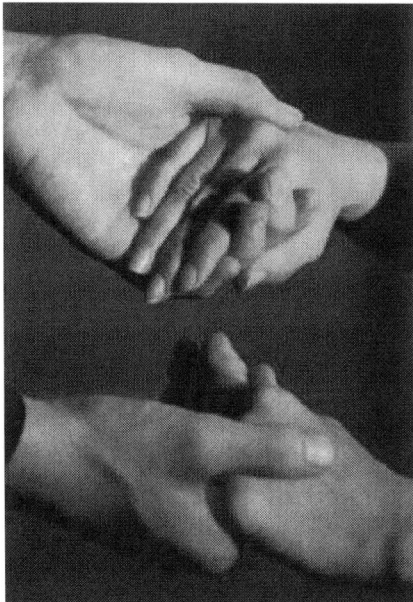

100
<u>Trace Any Problem To Its Cause</u>

If you're having a health issue or problem don't treat the symptoms. That may be fine to ease your pain but it won't cure what ails you. Finding the root cause is not an easy thing and in most cases you'll need to seek professional help. But its worth the effort. By treating the cause of a problem, rather than the symptoms, you'll become healthier. Rather than the problem just easing off then coming back at a later time, in the same or a different form, you can stop it dead in its tracks.

101
Be Adaptable

There is no need to go completely overboard with the information found in this book. If you can't to a certain thing, or eat a certain food you regularly do, you don't want to lose control over it and become stressed out. Also don't become militant in telling other people what they should or should not be doing. The healthier you are the more you will be able to break the rules on occasion without any ill effects. Just remember to make that the exception not the rule. You want to setup your lifestyle to be as healthy as possible. However being adaptable to your environment can be equally important. After all, adaptability is a hallmark of the human species.

Conclusion

There are two approaches to using the information found in this book and in any other source. You can do small steps at a time. Consistent and continual improvement. A single tip from here added to your life each day would make a huge difference over time. You can continually add (and subtract) as you work your way towards perfection. The other approach is to make massive changes fast. This can act as a jump-start, or a pivotal change in your life. Both approaches are valid. At times one may be better suited than another. The most important factor in both is that you take action. Now that you've finished this book do that. Take any one of these steps and do it right now. Reading this book alone won't make you healthy. All that matters is what you do with the information here. Take action NOW!

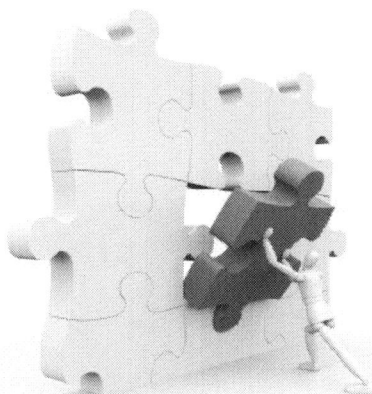

About The Author

Logan Christopher is the owner of Legendary Strength. He began training at the gym like everyone else during high school, getting programs out of the bodybuilding magazines because that was what he was exposed to. After more research he found out that there was a lot more out there from bodyweight exercises to kettlebells, hand strength to strongman lifts and more. He became an avid fan reading about and training with all these tools and different methods.

He's an avid fan of bodyweight exercises and got started with Matt Furey's Combat Conditioning even clinching the title of Combat Conditioning Athlete of the Year. To this day he continues with many bodyweight exercises, including hand balancing. He is also a certified Russian Kettlebell Instructor and performing strongman. Recent performances including pulling a fire truck by his hair.

His beginning foray into health was in search of not only maintaining a better quality of life, but seeking to enhance performance. With the loss of his mother to breast cancer he has began to delve further into health techniques and technologies and spreading that knowledge out to others.

<u>Websites by Logan Christopher</u>
www.LegendaryStrength.com
www.LostArtOfHandBalancing.com
www.KettlebellJuggling.com